How To Get Abs:

How to Get Abs Fast With An Extensive 6-Week Workout Plan

John Mayo

© 2015

Copyright/ Disclaimer Information

This book is not intended as a substitute for the medical advice of physicians. The reader should regularly consult a physician in matters relating to his/her health and particularly with respect to any symptoms that may require diagnosis or medical attention.

Table of Contents:

1) Introduction:

If you don't have to work hard for something, then it's usually not worth getting!

We all know why you're here, so let's get right down to it. First things first, congratulations for taking it upon yourself to flatten out your stomach. Abs and a flat stomach are probably the most desired aspect of the human body for a lot of people. Human beings will put themselves through immense pain at the gym, just so they can feel good about themselves when they take off their shirts. Can you really blame these people though? Let's face it; abs and a flat stomach look great and it's completely understandable that people want to achieve this look.

So who am I and why should you care? I'm the guy who's going to help you achieve your fitness goals. I'm a guy who has had abs for almost his entire life. I'm not being cocky about it; it's just a fact. I have been an athlete for my entire life and fitness is something that I take very seriously. I am a kayaking coach in Nova Scotia, Canada, and my passion is helping people increase their fitness level. Since abs are a very sought after thing, I really enjoy helping people flatten their stomachs and get ripped abs.

Let me be honest though, abs are not easy to get, nor are they easy to maintain. Anything in life that is worthwhile takes hard work and dedication to achieve and getting abs is no different. I have a theory about abs; I think that one of the main things that make abs so sexy is that when people see a flat stomach or ripped abs, they understand the hard work and self-discipline associated with this achievement. I think a lot of people view a person's stomach as a direct reflection of their personality, so when somebody has no belly fat, people generally think of that person as dedicated, focused and determined. Unless of course they cheated and got liposuction. Perhaps you think this theory is a stretch, but I believe it to hold quite true for most people.

So what makes this fitness book different from all the other "get abs fast" books out there? One word, honesty. I will not lie to you and tell you that at the end of this 6-week program you will have the chiseled abs and flat stomach that you've always desired. But if you take the information, workout techniques and fitness strategies that I am going to provide to you in the following pages, apply them continuously and never give up, you will undoubtedly get the results that you desire.

Make no mistake; this is going to be a difficult task. I talk a lot in my other fitness books about forming good habits. One you make something a habit, it becomes automatic and easy. The less you have to think about making good, healthy choices, the better off your life will be. This is why it is very important to get into good fitness routines and stick with them! That's where I come in. I am very good at getting people into healthy routines and creating manageable programs that will better their health. This specific book is obviously going to focus on how to get abs and if you follow along and do not stray from my program, I can almost guarantee that you will see results. Strap yourselves in, focus, tighten those abs up and let's get going!

2) Abs Behind the Scenes:

If you're going to ignore your eating habits completely and strictly focus on exercise, don't bother reading any further. Contrary to popular belief, diet is the MOST important factor for getting abs. It doesn't matter how many fantastic abdominal exercises you do everyday, if you're eating fatty, deep fried, over-processed foods, you're not going to see results.

-What I Try to Avoid:

Fried foods, white rice, bread, potatoes, cereal, beer/ liquid carbs, fatty sauces, trans fats (obviously), high fructose corn syrup (glucose- fructose in Canada).

* I consume every single thing listed above; I just try to consume very minimal amounts of each.

-What I Typically Try to Eat:

Quinoa & quinoa pasta, whole grain or multigrain bread (if I eat bread at all), avocadoes, kale, spinach, max 2-3 eggs a day, brown rice, ground flaxseed (frozen or refrigerated), chia seeds (great mixed with water), chicken breast, ground tomatoes (substitute for pasta sauce), bananas, natural peanut/ almond butter, dates, unsalted nuts and almonds, black beans, cliff bars, mixed vegetables, unsweetened almond milk, unsweetened coconut water/ oil, LOTS AND LOTS OF WATER!

If you only allow healthy food in your living space, it will make things a lot easier when you have a craving for something bad. Here are some meals you could make that I really enjoy:

Breakfast:

1) Large smoothie consisting of 1 banana, 4 dates, 1 tbs of natural peanut butter, 1 handful or kale/spinach, 1 tbs of ground flaxseed, 1 tbs of chia seeds, 1 tbs of coconut oil, 1 teaspoon of honey, lots of cinnamon, 1 handful of assorted frozen fruit, unsweetened almond milk and coconut water (add until there's a sufficient amount of liquid in the smoothie.)

2) 2 eggs and two pieces of toast. On the toast I like to put natural peanut butter, a little bit of honey and cinnamon.

3) Egg banana pancakes. 1 banana blended up with two eggs. Make just like you would pancakes. I like to add cinnamon and a touch of maple syrup.

Lunch:

1) Kale & spinach salad. Add avocado, chickpeas, ground flaxseed and black beans. For dressing I like to use a tiny bit of balsamic vinegar.

2) Pan fried haddock and a sweet potato with coconut oil.

3) Tuna sandwich on rye or flaxseed bread. I like to add lettuce, tomato and a bit of siracha sauce or pesto.

Dinner:

1) Spaghetti squash cooked in the oven. I like to add crushed tomatoes or a little bit of pesto.

2) Mango avocado salad. I use one mango and avocado, cut them up and add black beans, lettuce, jalapeños, quinoa, salsa and low fat corn chips. My personal favorite.

3) Mini pita pizzas. Add some pesto to pita bread with tomatoes, red pepper, onions and cheese. Bake the pita by the oven by itself first, add everything else and then put it back in the oven until the cheese melts.

The point I'm trying to make is that you need to take responsibility for your own diet. Keep in mind that diets should not be temporary. Your diet should be your lifestyle; you should make eating well a lifelong habit instead of a two-week fad. Temporary diets often lead to massive relapses in unhealthy eating. Lots of people start themselves out on unrealistic diets and never allow themselves to take a 'cheat day' and indulge in some tasty treats every once in a while. If you don't take a cheat day (I recommend once a week) you're sure to burn out and fail at your dieting plan.

Focus on your diet even harder than you focus on your exercises. If you get noting else out of this book please remember that no amount of abdominal exercise will get you a six pack/ flat stomach if you are eating like crap. Make no mistake, you will be strengthening your abs and getting a six pack if you eat like crap and workout like crazy, but I don't see much of a point in having abs if your stomach fat is covering it up. Your diet/ eating habits are key and you must not forget that!

3) * Fit Tip # 1:

Want to strengthen your core while you're at work, watching television or just sitting at home relaxing? Try to work on your posture every chance you get. By sitting up straight and consciously flexing your abs a little bit, in order to keep good posture, you are working your abs more than you know. While seated I also like to do what I call a 'flex set.' Here's what I mean:

- Flex your abs as hard and as fast as you can 20 times in a row

- Flex your abs and hold the position for 10 seconds, rest for 10 seconds and repeat 5 times

- Flex your abs as hard and as fast as you can 10 times in a row, Flex and hold for 60 seconds and then flex them hard and fast 10 more times

This can be done wherever you are because nobody can even tell that you're doing it. You could be in a meeting at work and do a quick flex set and nobody would even care. I also like to get my abs involved every time I stand up. Every time you stand you should consciously try to get your abs involved by flexing them hard during the entire process of standing up. Since you probably stand up a lot in the course of one day, you are forcing your abs to do a lot more work than they normally do. Once this becomes a habit, your abs will get a lot more use, which means they will get stronger and tighter!

4) Mixing it up:

I never lie on my back for twenty minutes and work my abs; I like to get more of my core involved because it's more fun and productive. There are more ways to work your abs than just the basic ab targeting exercises. I am a firm believer in functional strength, which essentially means that you strengthen your body as one unit, instead of doing isolated exercises like curls and crunches. I really enjoy circuit style workouts because they add an intense cardiovascular element to the workouts.

Many of the workouts that you are about to see in this 6-week training program are circuit-style workouts. In these circuits you will see exercises like; burpees, squats, pull-ups, lunges and jump rope/skipping. If you are unsure what these exercises are, I will explain them when the time comes. These may seem like unconventional exercises but I assure you they are vital if you want to achieve a strong and functional core.

Many of you are going to hate what I'm about to say, but cardiovascular training is an essential part of getting a flat stomach and toned abs. Cardiovascular training forces our body to sweat and burn fat, this exposes our abdominal muscles and flattens out our stomachs like nothing else. My favorite forms are cardiovascular training are running, skipping, swimming and kettle bells.

Kettle bells are my all time favorite piece of workout equipment. If you don't have own one or if you don't have access to one, fear not. Standard dumbbells can easily take the place of kettle bells. The only difference is that the weight isn't as effectively dispersed and they are harder to hold, but for our workout purposes, they will do just fine.

Remember, and this going for all workouts, once you feel the burn, KEEP GOING! If you give up as soon as you feel the pain, then you are wasting the crucial moments of your workouts. Abdominal pain is probably the worst burn you can get at the gym. Feeling like your core is about crumble beneath you is not a nice experience. But when you start to see results and you can feel that stomach starting to tighten up, all the pain will be worth it!

The good news is that once you follow this program and make core exercise a part of your daily routine, it will become much easier! The hard part is getting into the habit, but after six weeks of my program you will have no problem continuing on your own. Trust me, getting abs is a hell of a lot harder than maintaining them. While ab maintenance is still tough, it cannot compare to the difficulty of getting those abs to show for the first time.

5) Explanation of Key Exercises:

Here I will be explaining all of the exercises that you will have to do in the 6-week program. I will do my best to explain them all but if any of them seem unclear there are certainly YouTube videos out there that can give you a more in-depth idea on how to do particular exercises.

Understanding Workout Terminology:

When reading a workout the first number is the number of sets and the second number is the number of repetitions per set. So if you see 4 x 20, that means four sets of twenty reps per set. During a set you perform every exercise in order with no rest between exercises unless otherwise instructed. Some workouts will be timed such as 3 x 1:00, 1:00 off, 1:30 on. For this workout you would be doing each exercise in the set for one minute, resting for one minute and then doing that same exercise for one and a half minutes.

The Pushup:

Your stomach should be flat on the ground. Keep your arms at shoulder width apart, keep your back straight and make sure your chest touches the ground at the bottom and that your arms are straight at the end of every repetition.

The Kettle Bell Swing:

You can use dumbbells instead of kettle bells; it's just a little harder to hold onto them. Remember to start light, grip the kettle bell with two hands, let it swing between your legs, slightly bend your knees, then thrust your hips and straighten your legs while keeping your back straight to swing the kettle bell up to eye level. Arms should be slightly bent, feet at shoulder width apart. The weight you use is totally dependent on the number of repetitions you will be doing. If you are a beginner I recommend starting with 20-25 lbs. Your arms should not be doing much work at all, they are simply holding and guiding the kettle bell, the power of your swing should be coming from your legs, hips, core and back.

The Burpee:

Start in the standing position, jump down until your chest is on the ground, do a pushup keeping your back flat, jump your legs up into a squatted position and spring yourself up into the air with your arms reaching to the sky. With practice this movement will become fluid, but it remains a very challenging exercise.

The Squat:

Squats should be performed with your feet at shoulder width apart. Put your arms straight out in front of you and keep your back straight as you lower your bum to your ankles, keeping your legs parallel to one-another. Keep your back straight and keep your weight on your heels. Once you get as low as you can, use your legs to push yourself back up to the standing position, all the while keeping your back straight and your core tight

Jump Rope/ Skipping:

Make sure the skipping rope is the proper length. You can check this by holding the rope out in front of you, stepping on it with one foot and ensuring that the base of the handles comes up to at least your nipples. You can skip in a stationary position, or you can move around while skipping. Once you get good you can do some double unders (rope goes under you twice per jump), fast skipping, one leg skipping, heel skipping or side-to-side skipping.

The Pull-Up

Strict pull-ups are done straight up and down with your palms facing away from you. Do not swing or kip, you want to minimize the momentum and maximize the difficulty. I want you to only do strict pull-ups from now on. Get assistance if necessary when you're starting off, either from another person or by utilizing a weighted assistance mechanism found on certain pull-up machines.

The Mountain Climber:

Mountain climbers are great for your core. To perform, hover above the ground keeping your body horizontal. You should be on your toes and hands with your arms straight. One at a time, bring your knees towards your chest in an alternating motion. Every time both legs go in and out, you have completed one repetition.

Leg Lifts:

For leg lifts you want to lie flat on your back with your legs completely straight. Bring your legs up from the ground until they are at 90 degrees relative to your torso and then lower them until they hover above the ground. During the exercise you can either have your hands on the floor, or under your bum if you're finding the exercise difficult.

Squat Jumps:

Squat jumps are performed just like a regular squat, but you jump into the air about 1 foot upon extension of the legs.

Flexed Arm Hang (F.A.H):

Flexed arm hang is when you hang onto a chin-up bar with your arms bent and your eyes level with the bar. Stay up as long as the specified time says and if you lose your grip get right back up. This is a very difficult exercise.

The Reverse Crunch:

Reverse crunches are performed by lying flat on your back with your hands on the ground beside you. Your legs should be bent with your feet on the ground and you simply bring your knees up towards your chest and then back down to perform one repetition.

The Russian Twist:

For a Russian twist, sit down, lean back and let your legs hover above the ground. Rotate your core around side to side with your hands in front of you and your chest up. Let your hands touch the ground on either side of you to complete one full rep.

The Burpee Pull-Up

Burpee pull-ups are just like regular burpees, except for that when you jump up you need to grab a bar and do a pull-up at the end to complete a full rep. Use the momentum of your jump to assist you in your pull-up. You may find it easier to do the pull-up with one hand gripping the bar with your palm facing out, and one hand with the palm facing in.

The Plank:

 For a plank you want your stomach facing the ground. Put your elbows underneath your shoulders and lift yourself off the ground. Your weight should be on your elbows and your toes. Try to keep your back perfectly flat (don't sag your hips down to the ground or lift your bum really high into the air). Keep your abs tight and ensure that you have a comfortable base on your elbows/ forearms.

Leg Ins:

Leg ins are done from the plank position. Once in position, bring your right knee to your right elbow, and then back. Do the same with your left side and that equates to two reps.

Pikes:

 Pikes are also done from the plank position. Simply arch your back and stick your bum into the air, returning to the plank position to complete one repetition.

Flutter Kicks:

For flutter kicks you must lie on your back. Hover your legs above the ground and move them up and down as if you were kicking in the water. Up and down on each leg is one repetition.

U-Sits:

Sit on your bum with your knees bent and your feet hovering about one foot off the ground. The starting position for this exercise requires your legs to be straight (feet still hovering) and your arms should be straight, but off to the side as if you were trying to stop the walls from crushing in against you. To complete one repetition you must bend your knees up into your chest and clap your hands (arms remaining straight) in front of your knees.

The Super Burpee:

I want you to think 1 sit-up, 1 pushup, 1 burpee. I have dubbed this the super burpee because it is a superb exercise. Try to make this as smooth of a movement as you can. Do one complete sit-up, roll over onto your stomach and do a push up and then jump straight up into the air, like you would at the end of a regular burpee.

The Lunge Walk:

One leg at a time, step one foot out in front of you as far as you can, while dropping the opposite knee down to the ground (don't actually touch the knee on the ground, but get as close as you can). Get a nice smooth walking pattern going as you continue to switch legs.

The Sit-Up With Twist:

Keep your feet flat on the ground, knees pointed up to the sky and your hands touching your ears. Once you have fully sat up I want you to touch your right elbow to your left knee and then your left elbow to your right knee. This gets your abs a little more involved than a regular sit-up does.

Wall Sits: Put your back flat against a wall, bend your legs at about 90 degrees and hover above the ground like you

are sitting in an invisible chair. Hold the position for as long
as the specified time says.

Leg Ups: While holding onto a pull-up bar with your arms
straight, bring your knees up to your chest and flex your
abs.

6) *Fit Tip # 2:

Want to know a good way to wake your abs up in the morning? You don't need a gym, a bench or weights; you literally only need your own body weight to do this. It's really quite simple,

-Pick a good song that motivates you and pumps you up

-Try to pick a song that's between 3 and 5 minutes long (you will hate yourself if you pick a 10 minute song)

- Once you pick a good tune, find a comfortable area on the floor preferably with a rug or yoga mat.

- Play your song and then jump down onto the ground and into plank position.

- For a plank you want your stomach facing the ground. Put your elbows underneath your shoulders and lift yourself off the ground. Your weight should be on your elbows and your toes. Try to keep your back perfectly flat (don't sag your hips down to the ground or lift your bum really high into the air). Keep your abs tight and ensure that you have a comfortable base on your elbows/ forearms. If you want to make things easier you can move your feet wider apart. If you want to make things more difficult you can put your feet together. If you really want to make it more difficult you can wear a weight vest or a full backpack while doing your plank.

- Try to hold the plank for the entire duration of the song that you've selected. If you need to take a few breaks, that's totally fine, just make it through the entire song. This will be difficult for the first few mornings but in no time you will be selecting longer songs.

This is a good way to gauge the progress of your core strength/ endurance. The plank is a fantastic exercise because it forces your whole body to work together in fighting off gravity and keeping your stomach off the ground.

7) The 6-Week Training Schedule:

        Time to get down to the part you've all been waiting for. Remember to stick to a healthy eating plan while you're doing this 6-week program, or you're simply wasting your time. If you're finding things too easy at the start, feel free to add more sets or repetitions, as you feel necessary. Learning how to alter your workout program to fit your personal needs is an essential fitness skill. Remember to stick to the plan and never give up, the only thing that is going to get you the abs you've always wanted is focus and relentless persistence! I will explain any workouts that may not be clear to you

8) WEEK 1:

Monday:

3 sets of the following exercises. *Rest 2:00 between sets:

5 burpees

 20 mountain climbers

30 leg lifts

40 squats

Tuesday:

4 X 25 reps of:

Reverse crunches, leg lifts, leg ins, Russian twists, U-sits, flutter kicks.

*Rest 1:30 between sets

Wednesday:

3 X (3 minutes jump rope, 20 lunge walks, 3 minutes jump rope) *Rest 1:00 between sets.

Thursday:

4 X (1:30 plank, 1:00 rest, 1:00 plank)

Friday:

*No rest. 5 minutes of as many sets as you can complete of:

10 squats

 5 pushups

3 super burpees.

Saturday:

Run 15 minutes out, and then perform 30 squats, 20 mountain climbers and 10 burpees. Run 15 minutes back and then do 30 squats, 20 mountain climbers and 10 burpees. *No rest.

Sunday:

Rest day

Weekly Review:

If you have started to build a routine and stuck to these workouts in week 1, congratulations! You're on your way to a stronger core and a flat stomach. We are going to step up the intensity next week and you will find that the workout will continue to get harder in the weeks to follow. Before working out I advise that you warm-up by doing some dynamic movements such as; running on the spot, jumping jacks or even a couple minutes of jump rope. Static stretching should only be done once your workouts are complete.

"Excuses are like asses, everybody's got one, and they all stink."

- Anonymous

9) WEEK 2:

Monday:

3 sets of: 5 strict pull ups, 20 mountain climbers, 30 jumping jacks, 15 legs lifts

* Rest 2:00 between sets

Tuesday:

4 sets of 1-minute of burpees (do as many reps as possible in the one minute and rest for 2 minutes between sets)

Wednesday:

5 X 25 reps of: sit-ups with a twist, pikes, leg lifts, Russian twists, squats, kettle bell swings

* Rest 1:30 between sets

Thursday:

40 minute run, then 15 minutes of jump rope. * No rest

Friday:

Jump rope circuit, do double unders if possible. If you can't do double unders then do speed skipping for double the amount of jumps (Example: if you can't do 50 double unders then do 100 regular jumps as fast as you can). *No rest!

50 double unders, 50 jumping jacks

40 double unders, 40 mountain climbers

30 double unders, 30 leg lifts

20 double unders, 20 burpees

10 double unders, 10 pull-ups

Saturday:

2 x 1:30 on, 1:00 Rest, 1:00 on, of each exercise: squat jumps, plank, burpees, flutter kicks, kettle bell swings, mountain climbers. In each set you will be doing 1:30 and 1:00 of every exercise with 1:00 rest in between. You should rest 1:00 between exercises and 4:00 between sets.

Sunday:

6 x 4:00 jog, 1:00 sprint

You get no rest on this workout; once you finish the sprint you should jump right into your next four-minute jog. This is a fantastic speed/ endurance workout and it will get you sweating in a hurry.

Weekly Review:

At this point you should be fully into the routine of daily workouts. That was a tough week and it's not going to get any easier from here. Whenever you lose motivation, just imagine the next time you go to the beach. Do you want to be ashamed of your body, or do you want to be excited to get yourself into a bathing suit so that you can show off your hard work? The choice is up to you!

"Follow your passion, be prepared to work hard and sacrifice, and, above all, don't let anyone limit your dreams."

-Donovan Bailey

10) * Fit Tip # 3:

Is the only realistic time of day that you can complete your workouts in the morning? Are you always feeling tired and sluggish at this time of day? The following tip should help you wake up and feel ready to go at this tough time of day.

Have a shower before and after you workout. I'm not talking about a long and warm, relaxing shower; I'm taking about a quick cold shower.

-Simply get into the shower with the water at your normal temperature

- After one minute of warm water, switch the water to as cold as you can stand and let the water run down the back of your neck

- Try to control your breathing and do not panic

- Stay under the cold water for at least 1 minute and allow the water to touch every part of your body. Try to stay under the water for 3 minutes.

- Jump out of the shower, dry off and begin your workout

-Once your workout is done, jump back into another cold shower for at least three minutes. This should be easier since your body is warm from working out. After about three minutes turn the water back to warm for one minute, in order to regulate your body temperature, then get out of the shower.

Cold showers will wake you up in a hurry and studies also show that they can lead to weight loss. The cold water triggers shivering and shock, which has been proven to lead to weight loss. In his book "The 4-Hour Body," Tim Ferris actually cites one case in which a man lost over 40 pounds simply by using the cold exposure technique. Obviously this guy was taking things to the extreme, but still, it shows that cold showering can help you lose weight.

I personally don't take cold showers to lose weight. I take them to wake me up and to allow my body to feel alert, revitalized and ready for anything. I find them useful for strengthening mental fortitude. Resisting the urge of getting out of the shower, turning the water back to warm or breathing in a panicked way, takes an immense amount of will power.

This fit tip is pretty time consuming and if you don't have time for a full cold shower before your workout, I advise you to simply splash a bunch of cold water on your face before your workout, just to simply wake you up. This cold shower concept may seem ridiculous but trust me; cold showers will completely change how you feel. I've got many of my friends completely hooked on them and they are all benefiting greatly from this amazing technique.

11) WEEK 3:

Monday:

30 minute run. Then 3 x 1:30 wall sits, 50 mountain climbers, 100 jumping jacks. *No rest

Tuesday:

100 sit-ups
50 push ups
20 pull-ups
30 squats jumps
120 mountains climbers
50 burpees

(break the reps up in whichever way you want, just get it all done! Rest as needed but try to get it done as fast as possible.)

Wednesday:

4 x 5:00 jump rope, 1:00 F.A.H, 50 kettle bell swings
* Rest 2:00 between sets

Thursday:

2 x 1:00, 1:00 rest, 30 seconds on of each exercise: burpees, jumping jacks, push ups, plank, squat jumps, reverse crunches, kettle bell swings, lunge walks

Rest 1:00 between exercises and 2:00 between sets. You've completed one set once you've gone down the entire list and done a total of 1:30 of each exercise. Since we are doing 2 sets you must go down the entire list twice. In the end you will have completed 3:00 of each exercise.

Friday:

4 Sets of:

30 kettle bell swings

40 Russian twists

 30 leg lifts,

2:00 jump rope

1:30 plank

*Rest 2:30 between sets and don't rest between exercises

Saturday:

Rest

Sunday:

20 minute run, then

3 sets of:

10 burpees

20 reverse crucnches

1:00 plank

15 squat jumps

1:00 wall sit

5 pull ups

25 mountain climbers

*Rest 3:00 between sets and rest 15 seconds between exercises

Weekly Review:

That was the hardest week yet and if you made it through, I applaud you. You're halfway through this grueling workout program! Doesn't it feel great when your core starts to tighten up and you know your getting results?

"It does not matter how slowly you go as long as you do not stop."

-Confucius

12) WEEK 4:

Monday:

3 x 30 double unders, 30 lunge walks, 20 double unders, 20 pushups, 10 double unders, 10 burpees

(If you can't do double unders just do regular jump rope)

*Rest 2:00 between sets and don't rest between exercises

Tuesday:

4 x 50 kettle bell swings, 30 reverse crunches, 1:00 plank

* Rest 2:00 between sets and 20 seconds between exercises.

Wednesday:

1 hour run

Thursday:

3 X (2:00 plank, 1:00 rest, 1:30 plank)

* Rest 4:00 between sets

Friday:

5 X 2 minutes light skipping, 1 minute fast skipping. *No rest between sets

Saturday:

20 minute run, then:

2 X 5 burpee pullups, 15 pikes, 20 pushups, 30 flutter kicks, 40 jumping jacks, 10 leg ins, 3 super burpees

*Rest 3:00 between sets

Sunday:

Rest Day.

Try to complete 30 minutes of stretching during this rest day. Stretching consistently will help you to strengthen yours muscles and to prevent injury. Create a stretching routine that works for you and that you can complete regularly.

Weekly Review:

As I said before, cardiovascular training is an essential part of getting great abs and a flat stomach. At this point you should start to notice a great increase in your cardiovascular endurance. You have gone through some tough workouts that force your body to keep moving for a long period of time. If for some reason you are unable to run or if you hate it so much that you want to vomit, swimming laps is the best alternative. Swimming is, in my opinion, the best form of cardiovascular training on the planet. Many people don't have access to a pool, but if you do I suggest that you utilize it.

"Our greatest weakness lies in giving up. The most certain way to succeed is to always try just one more time."

-Thomas Edison

13) * Fit Tip # 4

Active rest is the only way to go! Throughout the 6-week workout plan you have seen me talk a lot about rest. When I say rest, I am not saying that you should flop down on the ground and relax until it's time to do your next set. You should NEVER be stationary during your rest time. Here's a breakdown of what I do during a rest session:

- Slowly walk around with my hands on my head, so as to open up my air passages

- Take long, slow and controlled breaths so I can prevent myself from cramping up.

- Take a small drink of water and splash water on my face

- Right before I start my next set I take a few deep breaths and mentally prepare myself for the next task

Rest is a vital part of your workout. If you are not properly utilizing your rest periods, your body will not be operating at its true potential. Some of the workouts I have given you do not have rest included in them. This is not an accident, these workouts are designed to increase your body's endurance and mentally strengthen you, so you will be able to push your body when it hurts the most. You will only ever truly enjoy rest after you have worked extremely hard!

14) WEEK 5:

Monday:

Complete as many burpees you can in 5 minutes! 40 reps is good. 50 reps is great. 75 reps is awesome. Anything over 100 reps is amazing!

Tuesday:

Complete 2:00 of every exercise. Rest 2:00 between exercises and make sure that you are completing as many reps as possible of every single exercise. Try not to rest at all during the 2 minute period of intensive exercise. The exercises are as follows:

Squat jumps, U-sits, jump rope (double unders if you can), mountain climbers, leg lifts, wall sits, jumping jacks, sit ups with twist, kettle bell swings, Russian twists

Wednesday:

Rest!

Thursday:

10 minutes of as many sets as you can complete of:

10 squats

5 pushups

3 super burpees.

Friday:

Total 40 minutes of running. During the 40 minutes you will stop every 5 minutes and perform 15 squats, 8 push-ups, 3 burpees.

Make sure you stop your watch timer while you are doing your exercise set and be sure to resume the watch timer when you begin running again.

Saturday:

8 X 10 pushups, 10 situps with twist, 5 burpees (No rest, complete this workout as fast as possible).

Sunday:

6 X 1:00 plank, 6 pull ups (30 seconds rest between sets)

Weekly Review:

You are turning into a workout machine! Keep up the great work because you are almost done the 6-week program. Take a moment to look back on some of the workouts you've been able to complete over the past 5 weeks and give yourself a pat on the back.

"The starting point of all achievement is desire."

-Napoleon Hill

15) *Fit Tip # 5:

Struggling to finish those last few repetitions? Are you finding that you are utterly drained during your workouts? Dehydration is a major contributing factor to exercise fatigue. If you don't have enough water in your body, you will not be able to function at an optimal level, especially when you are sweating!

So how much water is enough water? Honestly, you can never really have too much, unless of course you're drowning. I suggest drinking a lot of water before your workout, at least 600ml (about 20 ounces).

Cut back your water intake during your workout to avoid having a sloshing feeling in your stomach. During your workouts I advise only taking small mouthfuls of water every 5-8 minutes.

After your workout is complete and your body has released a ton of water in the form of sweat, it's time to drink a TON! Well not literally a ton, but I advise drinking at least 1200ml if you sweat a lot during your exercises.

I also advise splashing water on your face to cool yourself down. Did you know that as soon as your face is hit with cold water your heart rate begins to slow? This is called the 'mammalian diving reflex.' It happens because your body is preparing to survive underwater without oxygen for as long as it can. By slowing your heart rate and the flow of blood, your body is able to survive longer without air. Keeping your heart rate in check is an important part of working out, so splashing cold water on your face during workouts is a fantastic idea. This is another reason why cold showering is a great idea.

Carrying a water bottle with your throughout the day is one of the best things you can do, and your body will thank you for it by offering you better performance during your workouts. Every time you pass a water fountain you should take a drink and if you're carrying a water bottle with you, I advise taking a small drink every time the thought crosses your mind.

16) WEEK 6:

Monday:

15 minutes of as many sets as you can complete of:

10 squats

5 pushups

3 super burpees.

Tuesday:

10 X 2:00 jog, 1:00 sprint, 1:30 rest. (Keep yourself moving the whole time. Even on the rest you should be walking slowly. Run as fast as possible during the 1:00 sprint!)

Wednesday:

Jump rope circuit, do double unders if possible. If you can't do double unders then do speed skipping for double the amount of jumps (Example: if you can't do 50 double unders then do 100 regular jumps as fast as you can).

Do 2 X the following circuit: (rest 3:00 between sets)

50 double unders, 50 mountain climbers

40 double unders, 40 jumping jacks

30 double unders, 30 leg ins

20 double unders, 20 pikes

10 double unders, 10 leg ups

Thursday:

Rest!

Friday:

25 minute jog

Saturday:

5 x 30 reps of:

kettle bell swings

squats

reverse crunches

lunge walks

*Rest 2:00 between sets

Sunday:

The Kamikaze:

4 Sets of:

20 burpees

30 kettle bell swings

10 pull ups

30 lunge walks

50 squats

1:30 plank

30 mountain climbers

20 U-sits

15 reverse crunches

20 Russian twists

*Rest 5:00 between sets

Weekly Review:

You've done it, great work! If you have followed this program religiously and stuck to a healthy diet, then I have no doubt that you are enjoying some fantastic results. That program was far from a walk in the park, I know because I myself have done every single one of the workouts that you just completed. Many of them are extremely difficult and require an immense amount of dedication to get through.

"When you want to succeed as bad as you want to breathe, then you will be successful."

-Eric Thomas

17) Conclusion:

This is a pivotal moment in your life. You now have the information required to change your lifestyle and your body forever. The question remains; will you use this information to better your life? Or will you make excuses and not take action? If you want to live a happy life, you have to be a doer. You must attack every aspect of your life with a ferocious, never quit attitude. If you apply this attitude to every aspect of your life, then there is no way you can be unsuccessful.

I've heard many people in my life say,

"Nobody actually enjoys working out, what people truly enjoy is the positive influence working out has on their body."

Yes and no. I obviously enjoy how by body looks when I stick to a strict workout schedule but I also love the total equilibrium that it brings to every other dimension of my life. By pushing yourself during a workout, you're getting your body and your mind used to NEVER QUITTING at anything in life. This attitude will carry over into other aspects of your life and make you a truly remarkable and unstoppable human being. By staying in control of your body during a workout you also learn how to stay in control of your life. I notice a direct correlation between my mood and my workout schedule. If I'm not sticking to my workout plan, then I feel horrible.

Previously in 'Fit Tip # 2' I mentioned doing the plank exercise to your favorite song. This is one of my preferred forms of exercise because it exemplifies the power of your mind. Planking is such a simple exercise because all you have to do is fight off the relatively weak force of gravity. You just have to keep your body flat and your stomach off the ground, but as the seconds tick, this becomes increasingly difficult. 1 minute in you feel okay, 2 minutes in things start to hurt, 3 minutes in you want to quit, and it continues.

The point here is that planking is only as hard as you make it. If I plank for twenty seconds and you plank for four minutes, there is simply no comparison between the levels of difficulty we are both experiencing. I like to compare life to planking, because it's really only as hard as you make it. Obviously there are exceptions and people get dealt really crappy hands in life, but for the most part I believe that people control their own success. If you are willing to commit to something in life and fight for it, you can do it, it really just depends on how long your are willing to stay strong for, how long can you keep your body planked? How long can you keep your stomach off the ground until it feels like your abs are ripping apart? Are you willing to keep persisting until your muscles begin to twitch and your soul begins to tremble?

You're only as strong as your willpower. Human beings are capable of phenomenal things if they apply their minds properly. Many people used to believe that since we didn't have wings we would never be able to fly. We certainly solved that problem and now you are going to solve the problem of not having a flat stomach and great abs. It all starts with desire and willpower, if you want it bad enough and you don't give up, it will be impossible for you to fail.

18) My Sincere Thanks:

Congratulations and thank you for taking the time to read this book. I hope this book has been helpful to you and that you get the results you are looking for. Check out some of my other titles on my Amazon author page and contact me directly at any time if you have any questions about any of the material in my books. Keep your eyes open for my next "How to Get Abs" book which will be coming out in the near future!

johnmayo@hotmail.com

Made in the USA
Middletown, DE
01 September 2019